Penis Exercise

The Complete Penile Fitness System

By Nate Hawking

Contents

Chapter 1. Introduction

You *can* maximize the girth, length and size of your penis through exercises. "Oh sure," you're probably thinking, "just like a million of those spam emails that promised results while charging exorbitant prices through a website that looked like it was put together by a first year computer science student".

It's a valid point. The penis enlargement industry has been overrun by scammers, crooks and false experts who don't know what they're talking about, all out to make a quick buck.

Fair enough, that penile cream you ordered probably contained no special ingredients and the results were less than miraculous, to say the least. So, how is this book different? Why is it that a hundred other products offering results never deliver but this might work somehow?

Well, inspired by the success of my Talking Dirty book, I decided to take my knowledge of the various penis exercises and construct a no nonsense fitness system using similar philosophy. That philosophy is to cut to the chase, eliminate wordiness and empty phrases and instead focus on the exercises that deliver results. *Zero* filler. It's always my aim to say more with less so while this won't be the longest book you read on the subject I did all I could to make sure it would be the best.

But I digress. I was having a conversation with a friend who had come across a website that stated that the average penis size was between eight and nine inches when erect. Now, I know for a fact that this isn't true since I'm very aware of the true statistics involving size. Who would say something so blatantly ridiculous? I had him show me the website, and I scrolled through their so-called 'facts', and right there on the top there was the claim.

This wasn't all it had to say. According to this website, 85% of women fake their orgasms due to their man being too small, and that a healthy male can have up to three orgasms in an hour. Apparently, anyone who did not see these results was somehow defective, and should rush to buy their product immediately to remedy the situation. Just another advertisement for a sham penis enhancing cream.

This probably won't come to a shock to anyone, and it certainly didn't to me. I had heard of this product several times in the past, not only online, but in magazine articles, on television commercials, and even on drug store shelves. It's like a hundred other products created by someone without an ounce of real knowledge on the topic. In short, it is packaged hope, one that might make you wonder: How many men actually buy into this crap?

Apparently, enough men to make penis enhancers one of the most popular selling items in the industry. But I didn't address the main question yet. That question is how is this book different?

This book is different in that we don't offer revolutionary claims, miraculous promises or quick fix solutions. The main premise of this book is the size, girth and the overall performance of your male organ can be optimized through a specific set of exercises developed by me over years of research, both primary and secondary.

Will this work for everyone? Well, there is no such thing as a product that works equally well for everyone. Will it not work for some? Yes, but it should be very few. Will it for most? I think so. Regardless of an exercise program, people will make varying progress based on their natural ability, proper exercise application, regular exercising, etc. So, while I can't claim that your penis will double in size as a result of these exercise, I think this book will contain exercises everyone can apply to improve their sexual performance.

So, how will we get there? We'll analyze the real facts about size and performance. We'll analyze all of those penis creams and quick fix solutions that don't work. But, most importantly, I will introduce a set of exercises I refer to as Nate Hawking's Complete Penile Exercise System, which target all areas of your organ from length, girth, hardness, all the way to performance.

And don't worry; we won't use any nutty holistic remedy recipes with ridiculous claims about the use of rhino horn, and waving your erection at a full moon to give it the power of the night. Everything provided here will objectively address pills, various devices, and even surgery, as well as teach you about the exercise system that may work without resorting to more extreme measures. And the best part: the only equipment you'll need is your penis, and your hands, which I am guessing you are already quite used to combining. Don't bother denying it!

We will start with some cold, hard (pardon the pun) facts:

1). The average penis size varies by country, but the most commonly seen statistics are between 5.75 inches, and 6.25 inches long.

2). The average male can perform sexually once a day to once every other day, which may include masturbation.

3). There are two different kinds of penis, each one with its' own change of proportions during erections. The first is a penis that lengthens during an erection. The second is one that stays approximately the same size, and just hardens. Neither is better than the other, and there is rarely a different in size when both erect.

4). Virginity can affect penis size. The difference in testosterone levels actually shifts dramatically after a man has sex for the first time. If you virgins are worried about the size of the jimmy, don't worry. You will probably notice a difference once you have broken him in.

5). Medical conditions and health factors may affect the size of your penis. Anything that effects blood flow can make a difference in the size, look, and performance, as a matter of fact. Not only does this mean heart conditions or high blood pressure.

Smoking or drinking too much is often an issue men don't associate with their penile problems.

This, folks, is the truth that those penis enhancement manufacturers don't want you to know. You might be thinking "Hey, that means I am normal," and you would be right in that assumption. But the fact that you are seeking this book out in the first place shows that you aren't happy with 'normal'. Who wants to be average? There is always room for improvement, and if you really want to wow your partner, potential partner, your next one night stand, or just yourself, you can work towards something bigger and better.

I am going to teach you how to do that, and it shouldn't take more than a few minutes a day but you will need to do these exercises on a regular basis. Not only that, but it will be easy, painless, and you should notice progress within a few weeks. This is a process that anyone can aim for, and with few risks involved. Well, unless you consider the stalker tendencies of the next person you sleep with to be a risk, in which case you will want to forgo any further reading and stay just the way you are.

The process will go in small steps for you to follow for as long as it takes for you to find yourself satisfied.

First, you will find out about making your own workout regimen. This will mean looking honestly at what you have, and what you will want to work on. Are you worried about your length? Do you think you could be a little thicker? Is it the hardness or number of erections that has you feeling antsy? It could be all three. Or maybe you just want to enhance the overall performance, stamina, or distance of your ejaculation. You can even work to create greater pleasure in your orgasms.

Next, you will learn the different exercises that will help you to achieve everything you worked out in the first step. This includes learning how often to do them, how many times, and for how long. You will also find out what not to do. After all, too much of a good thing can be harmful, and the last thing you will want is to yank it off in an attempt at improvement. Ever heard of a penile sprain? Take it from me, it's not an experience you want to do more than read about.

Last, you will find out about what doesn't work, and the truth about enhancers. It goes beyond just not working. Some will work for a time, and then stop. Some will actually cause damage to the penis, or the body as a whole. Some will empty your bank account, and for such little results that you might as well have bought a sports car and been done with it.

That is what this book is all about, and I am here to guide you through it all. So strap in, get ready, and get ready for some real results. Any puns and corny jokes along the way are a byproduct, and I apologize in advance. I promise you it will be worth listening to me when you look down one morning and realize the work was worth it.

Chapter 2: The Complete Penile Fitness System

Now that you know that it is possible to add a bit of pep to your step, it is time to find out how. The Complete Penile Fitness System is my own personal method of maximizing the performance of your sexual organ. Through this system you will learn all you need to know to do everything from lasting longer to maximizing the length to girth of your penis. Hopefully, in the end you will have the penis that you have always wanted, both for your and your partner's satisfaction.

Now before you ask, I am going to answer a question several people have already brought up: Have I tested the Complete Penile Fitness System on myself? While I would love to be able to tell you that I am the man with the uber schlong, and that I have never had a moment of doubt about my size and performance, I can't. I, like so many others, was not completely satisfied with every aspect of my sexual performance. And impressing my wife was a part of me wanting to work on my game so to speak.

So, the short answer is: yes. I have used these exercises myself, and used my experienced to develop the best possible exercise routine, in my experience. Many of these exercises are prescribed for this or another reason, but I found the perfect combination that worked for me as well as for others. So, there is no good reason of why it wouldn't work for you.

How Does the Complete Penile Fitness System Work?

The concept behind this set of exercises is deceptively simple. The exercises provided in this book are meant to provide internal traction. Using your hand, you will perform a number of movements, such as slapping, pulling, twisting, and other workouts that can sound a lot more painful than they actually are. As you do this, the penile tissue should become more flexible, agile and more prone to expand. This tissue is often referred to as the corpora cavernosa.

Think of the corpora cavernosa as the 'chambers' of the penis. These sections are where the blood flows when it becomes erect. The more blood that is held in these chambers, the bigger and harder you're going to get. Expanding the tissue makes these chambers more agile, allowing for more blood flow, and – yep, you guessed it – a better performing, harder, bigger penis. Doesn't sound like rocket science, right?

How is This Different from a Penis Traction Device?

Those of you who have looked online for enhancers have probably heard of those traction devices. These are medical instruments used mostly for men with a severe penis curvature, or a condition known as micro-penis syndrome (try to guess what that entails). The device is placed on the penis in order to stretch out the tissue, creating more space within the chambers in much the same way that penis exercises do.

Now, this may seem like the same thing, but it is actually a little more different than you might think. First of all, the way the mentioned device is designed is to apply traction externally. The movement that it creates can only expand the corpora cavernosa from the outside. This is different than The Complete Penile Fitness System, which, despite being applied externally, actually provide internal traction as well. Due to the specific physical nature of the exercises both of the above areas are targeted thereby providing better, long lasting results.

Secondly, those devices are fairly expensive, and rarely do they guarantee results so the cost to results ratio is high. Also, most of them are available only through a prescription, and even then only to a small percentage of men who have a "serious problem", as determined by the doctor. Then there are those over the counter products. Well, I am sure most men have tried at least one of those and I can attest myself that the results from those can vary from underwhelming to downright disappointing.

How Many Exercises Will I Need to Learn?

This will depend on you and your individual goals. Several of the workouts are designed for more than one purpose. This means you will only have to learn one for two different aspects, or more if you want to bulk up those gains a little more. You will have to learn several if you wish to gain length, girth, increased hardness, and better stamina, for example.

How Often Will I Need to Do These Exercises?

Each workout should be performed for no more than 10 – 15 minutes a day so the time commitment is minimal. Some systems suggest longer, usually around 30 minutes a day, but in my experience, this is suboptimal. Furthermore, some of the mentioned exercises can be somewhat demanding so practicing for half an hour everyday can be downright dangerous. Remember: less is often more. I realize you want to work on your penile fitness, but I am assuming one of those improvements doesn't entail yanking it off completely. So remember: pace yourself and don't overdo it, especially if you have to perform with your lady that same evening.

How Long Until I See Results?

Different men see results in different times. My own experience had me seeing an increase in size in just a little over two and a half weeks. The results on my stamina began in just a few days more, and by the noticeable size difference can vary vastly depending on build, complexion and genetics. You should notice improvement in the time period between seven and ten days, with drastic changes occurring closer to the ten day phase.

Now, with all of this in mind, I don't want you walking away from this chapter thinking that if you keep it up you will end up with something the size of an arm dangling between your legs. I have never seen anyone with more than a three inch increase, and most started out on the smaller side to begin with. You will see significant changes, but don't expect miracles or quick fixes.

But, if you are looking for reasonable improvements, get ready to work hard and low and behold, your sex life will take a turn for the better. If these exercises are performed as specified, you stick to the schedule and neither overdo or under do them, you should experience the following improvements: better orgasms, stronger ejaculations, better stamina, control and agility of your male organ.

So, if you are tired of reading about it, and you are ready to get started, read on. Your sexual life won't wait and no one else will do this for you so let's take this matter into our own hands, so to speak.

Chapter 3: Developing Your Exercise Plan

Now we come to the 'hard' part: (see what I mean about puns?) creating an exercise routine. Many penis exercise programs do not address this properly, which I believe is a mistake. Instead of enabling you to create a unique system that will yield the greatest gains, they start you off with a one-size-fits-all booster plan. Once that plan is over, they put you on another, which may or may not target what you are looking to improve.

I don't know about you, but to me that hardly seems like the way to go. What good is a routine that is made to give you length, when you are worried about girth? What good is a program concerned with adding girth, if all you need is more sexual control? If you don't care about size so much but always come too soon, why would you want to do a program targeted at people with completely different goals? There is no point in spending weeks working towards a goal if it's not a goal that you personally have defined.

Coming up with a routine can be difficult because it means you have to look at yourself, and your penis, honestly, which is something that men everywhere seem to have a great deal of trouble doing. What's more, the digital age has made us even more reluctant to admit the truth. When was the last time you entered into a chatroom and told the 40-year-old man pretending to be a woman that you were chatting with that you had an average penis of about five-and-a-half inches? Chances are, you gave a slightly ridiculous measure of nine or ten inches, and why not? Of course she told you she was a platinum blonde with double D breasts but I digress.

Anyway, the point is, it is time to give up the lying and face the hard (another one!) facts.

Step One: What Have I Got?

Take real stock of what you want to change, and what you feel you're happy with. Let's say you have a length of six inches, and you are happy with it. But you have always worried that you might be just the slightest bit on the thin side, and you want to change that. You would add 'girth' to the list of exercise requirements in your routine.

Next, you will want to look at performance, and this is where it can get a little tricky. Most men don't want to admit they may have a problem here, whether it is with premature ejaculation, frequency of erections, or just the ability to keep it up. If you honestly don't have a problem, do you think you could at least improve? Do you want better stamina, stronger orgasms, and ejaculations that shoot further? Then add these to your list of workout priorities.

Alright, by now you've already taken a moment to be honest with yourself about your performance. And that's a great start; you've just done what few men actually find themselves able to do. You're ready for the second step.

Step Two: What is Available?

Now, we will talk about the various exercises you can include in your routine. There are several different types, and for several different purposes. However, some will target more than one area, such as length and girth, or stamina and control. When this occurs, I will put the exercise into the most common area for its use, and then make a small note letting you know what else it may affect.

The main exercises used in The Complete Penile Fitness System will include:

• Power Stretch

• V Stretch

- Circular Stretch

- Jelq Form 1

- Jelq Form 2

- Jelq Form 3

- Jelq Form 4

- Sit Down Stretch

- Kegels

- Sit Down Wally Ups

- Flex Ups

Step 3: What Tools (Besides My Own) Do I Need?

I know, I know, I said you wouldn't need anything but the well known combination of your penis and your hand. Well, you actually will need just a few other things for some of the exercises; the good news is those are very easy to come by. Having those items will make these exercises go smoother, and in the end maximize the achieved results. Luckily, they cost very little, or maybe even nothing at all, as I would assume you would have these lying around the house somewhere.

• Hot water.

Don't worry, I'm not suggesting that you should scald your penis in a boiling pot, or anything sadistic. But having hot water around when doing these will help increase the blood flow, as well as relax the tissue to optimize expansion. As such, doing this in a hot shower or bath is a good idea.

Make sure it isn't too hot, you don't want to scald yourself now. It just has to be warm and comfortable, like any shower of bath would be. If you prefer, you could always just use a heating pad, hot, wet rag, or even a bowl of warm water for dipping if you like. As long as you get heat to your penis, and make it more malleable.

• Lubricant

You will need something to smooth the way, whether you are circumcised or not. This doesn't have to be anything fancy, or even something like KY. It just has to be gentle on the skin, and water soluble, like anything you might use when you are all alone, and maybe a little lonely (you know exactly what I'm talking about).

Some popular choices are lotion, conditioner, or Vaseline. I would recommend the later, as it is thick, and it doesn't rub off easily. It also won't wash off with the use of hot water, and so you don't have to keep reapplying.

That's it. You don't need anything else to get started, and if you have these things you can jump into your routine right away. I would recommend keeping track of what exercises you use by writing them done, and regularly measuring your progress along the way. That way, you will be able to watch your results as you begin to grow.

If you are ready to get started, let's begin!

Chapter 4: Length Exercises

One of the most common reasons for penile enhancement has to do with length. That isn't surprising, not if you consider the fact that penis size is almost always measures purely in inches of length. You rarely hear about girth, and even less about stamina, when talking about the shape of a man's unit. This may or may not be fair, but I am not here to argue ethics with you. I am here to help you maximize your penis length, so you can stand back at the urinal with pride.

Each one of these exercises can be done alone, or implemented into a longer routine. Just remember that if you are going to use multiple exercises within this category, added to others, you have to compensate for the time. The entire routine should not exceed the ten to fifteen minutes. Each rep should be done within a matter of seconds, with several reps in one exercise. You will probably do approximately a hundred movements her exercise.

The Warm Up

Before doing any exercise, you should begin by warming yourself up. This is meant both literally and figuratively. As mentioned before, you should use a heating pad, warm water, and a warm room...anything that will increase the blood flow through the tissue. The blood has to be pumping, and so for many you have to be in a semi-erect, or erect state. How you choose to do this will be up to you. Some will have to be done while flaccid. I will note this in the exercise.

Once you have reached that state, slowly begin to rub the shaft in gentle circle, moving from the base up to just under the head. Do this up to five times, until the skin is slightly more sensitive. This should not end in orgasm, so if that starts to feel a little too good, you need to stop. If you end up getting off, you won't be getting into the routine, got me?

The Power Stretch

Standing with your feet a shoulder width apart, place your thumb and forefinger on either side just under the head of the penis. Begin to stretch it as far as it can go without becoming painful, directly in front of you. This should feel slightly straining, but should never actually hurt. If it hurts, then reduce the stretch slightly. There are no points here for tearing your member off. Next, take a deep breath and tense your PC muscles (in other words, clench your butt, thighs, and abdomen). Hold for five seconds, and then slowly release your muscles as you put your penis back to its' normal length. You will notice your penis becoming more flushed with color, especially at the head. This is normal, and desired. The Power Stretch is further illustrated on the next page.

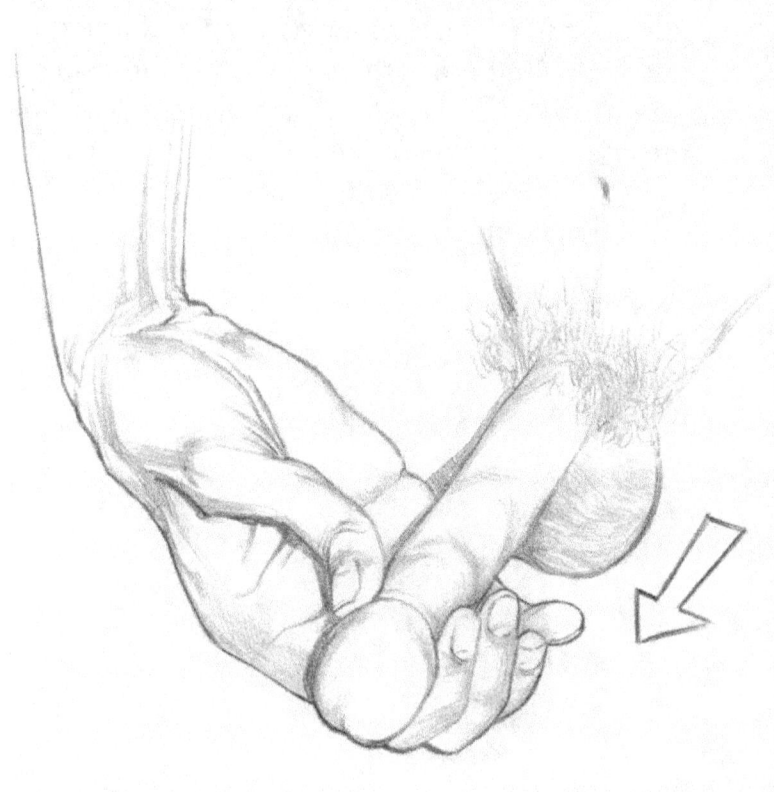

The Sit Down Stretch

This exercise is actually done better when in a closer-to-flaccid state. It is also the only exercise that you can do for longer than the ten to fifteen recommended minutes. Standing up, hold your penis in the same way as with the Power Stretch, with your thumb and forefinger holding just under the head. Slowly stretch it out as far as you can without causing pain. Then, pull the penis underneath you, so that it lies along the perineum (in other words, the skin between your balls and your anus). Slowly sit down in a firm chair, keeping your penis in place. This will add length when flaccid, though not necessarily when erect.

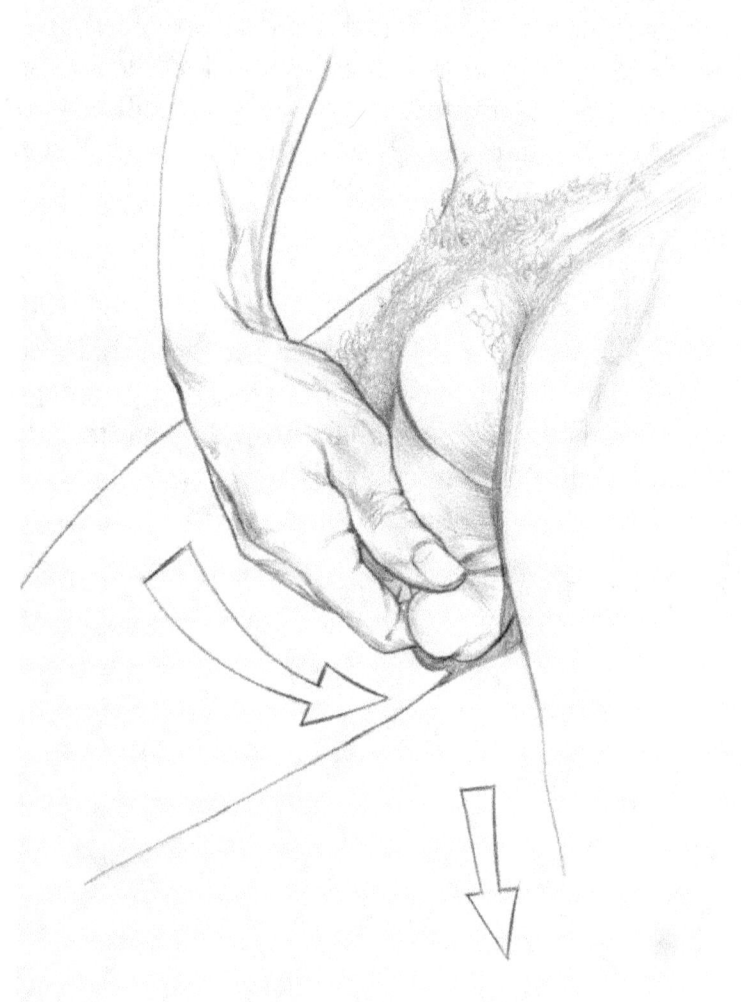

The V Stretch

While fully flaccid, stretch the penis out as far as it can go with one hand. You may want to use a cloth to do this, in order to keep the hand from slipping. Slowly use your other hand to grip the middle of the shaft between to fingers. Using the hand that was stretching, slowly bend the penis into a 'V' shape. Do this in first on direction, then another, and so on until you have done it in every direction it can be bent easily. Hold for five seconds each time. When you are done, slowly release back into the stretch, and then into its' natural position. Never try to do this when erect, or even semi-erect. I don't think it is much of a leap of the imagination to figure out why.

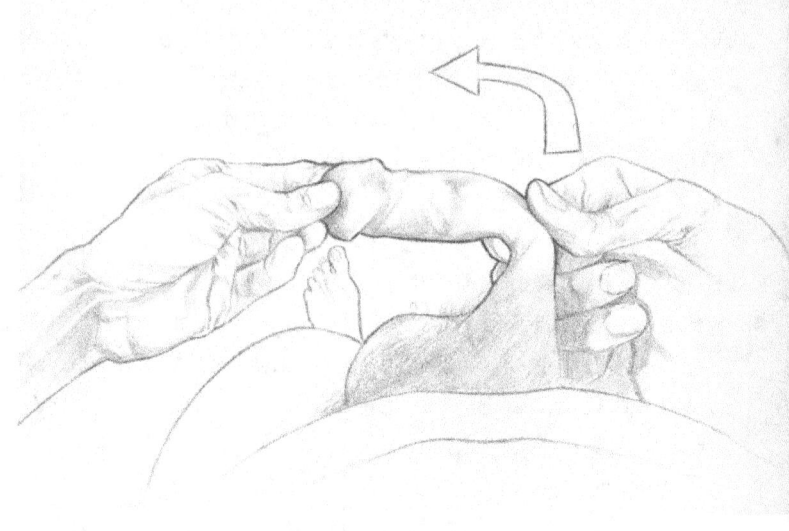

The Circular Stretch

Stretch the penis out in front of you as far as it can go and hold for approximately five second. Slowly release it back into its' usual position without actually letting go of the head. Do this once more, only don't release it, just hold it out in front of you for another five seconds. Once this is done you may slowly begin to rotate the penis in a wide, circular motion. Make sure it is a slow, proper circle, taking around three to five seconds per rotation. If this is painful, use a smaller circle, but keep in mind that the wider it is, the deeper into the tissue the blood will flow.

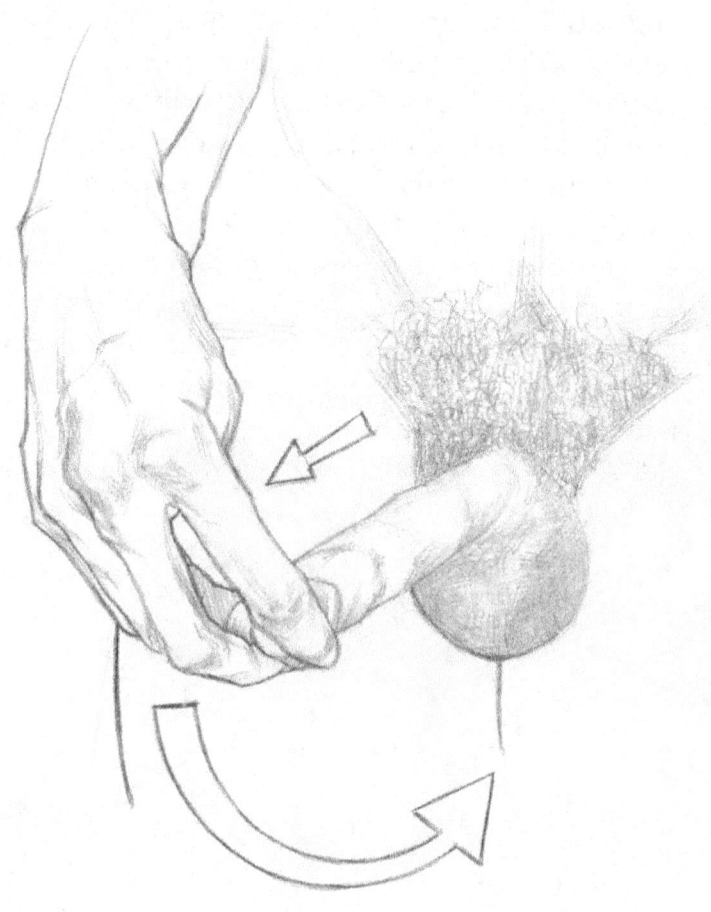

Now, before we move on to the next set or workouts, let me make one thing perfectly clear now: These will not begin working immediately! I cannot tell you how many emails, letters, phone calls, and comments I have gotten from men who started using the exercises I recommended, and within 24 hours were complaining about their Johnson not magically sprouting five inches. Look, these should work, but they take a little longer than a day or two for you to notice the change.

As I stated before (but will state again for those of you who have skipped straight to the workouts), these will usually take ten to fourteen days before you start to see effects. Have a little patience, and keep it up. In the end it will be worth it.

Chapter 5: Girth Exercises

Conduct the warm up provided in Chapter 4. If you are doing this as a larger part of a routine, do a gentle warm up in between these and the others. Once you are ready to begin, make sure the room is warm, and that you are semi-erect for the duration of these various jelquing exercises. Make sure that you use plenty of lubrication for all girth routines to reduce chaffing. You don't want to end up explaining to your partner about a rash, do you?

Jelq Form 1

Starting from the base of the penis, wrap your thumb and forefinger around your semi-erect penis. Push downwards and out, holding tightly so that blood rushes up towards the head. Hold for four seconds then release, moving up slightly just above the base of the shaft. Repeat the movement, holding four seconds each time as you make your way up. You should notice the head becoming more and more red, and over the course of a few weeks you will see a significant increase in head size, as well as in the overall girth of the shaft. Next page will illustrate how to do this

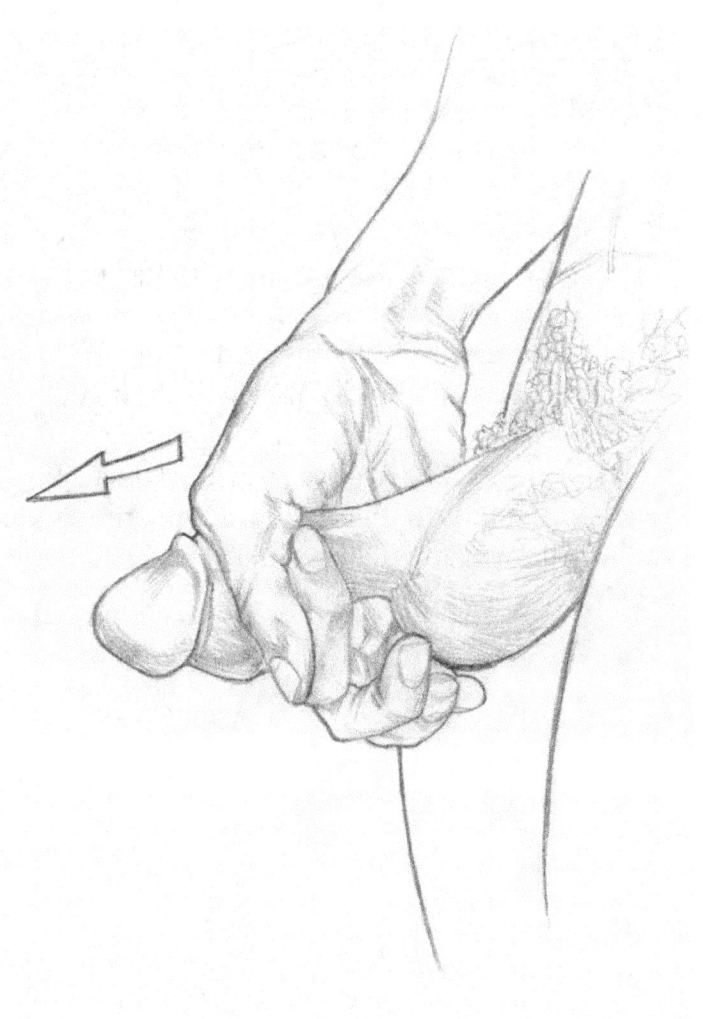

Jelq Form 2

This jelq is more or less the same as above, only you will be alternating hands, and begin on a flaccid penis. As the penis becomes more erect due to stimulation, apply more pressure as your hands move down in a 'milking' motion. Because you are starting off in a flaccid state you can apply more strokes than with other methods. You don't have to hold it for the four seconds, instead moving immediately to the other hand, one after the other, in slow but steady strokes down. Once you have reached the base with one hand, the other should be making its' way down as well.

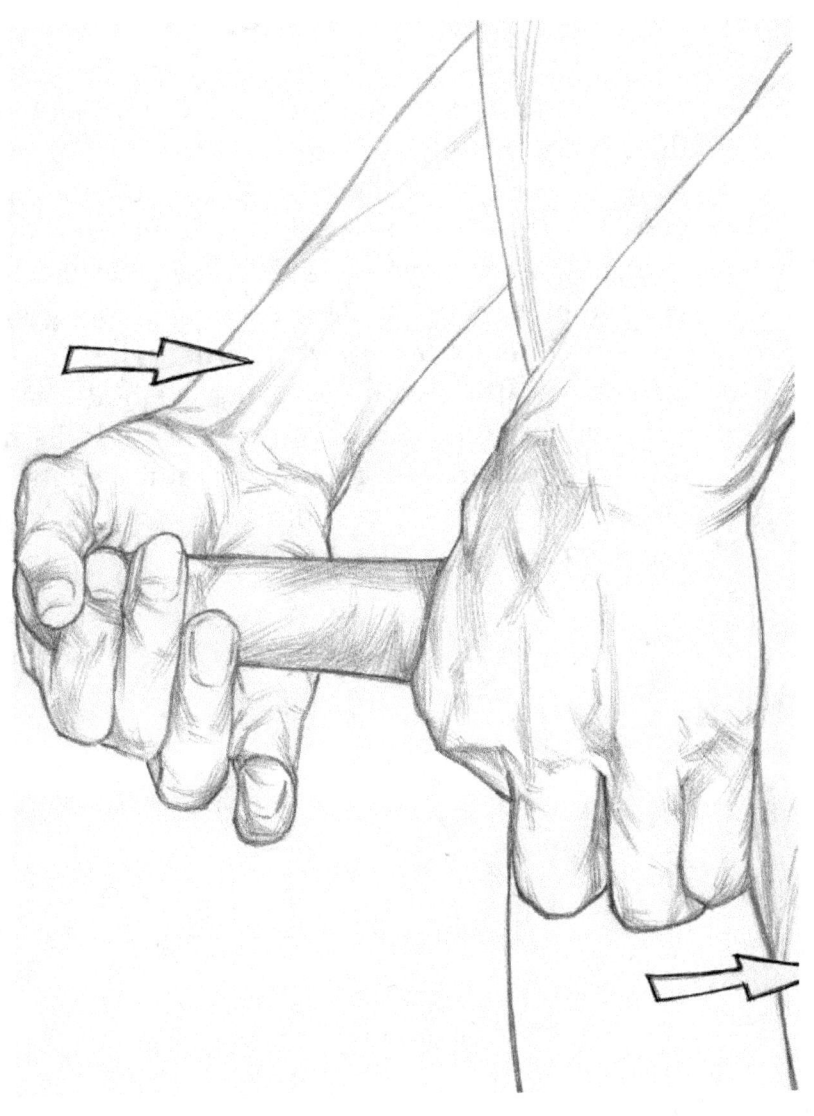

Jelq Form 3

This is often considered the method that will bring the fastest results, though not the most drastic. Gripping the base of the penis as before, rub upward towards the head, firmly pressing down and stretching as you go. Once you approach the head, use the other hand to do the same, stroking in the same way, one hand after the other. This is a little different than the other milking methods, as it is more rapid, and the way you press should be more firm, the skin stretching along the entire length. This might be slightly uncomfortable, but shouldn't actually hurt.

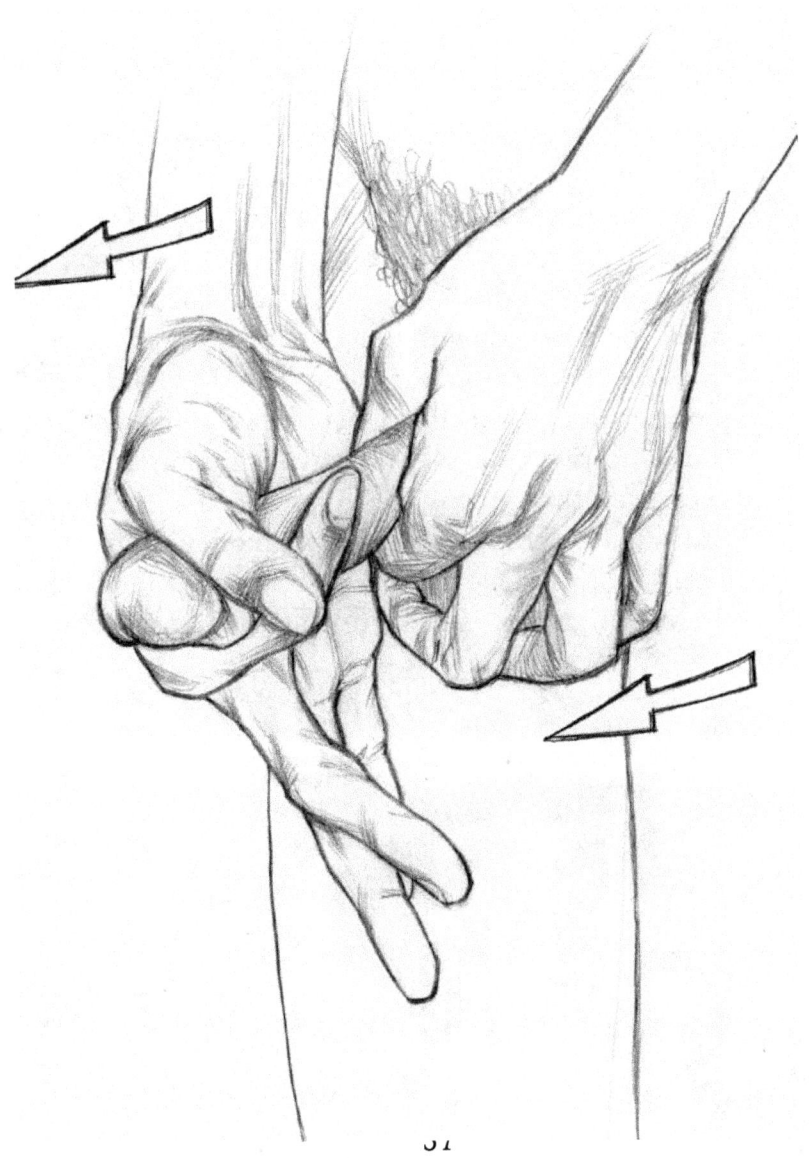

Jelq Form 4

This is known as the Tao method, and it is a well known one from those who frequent forums and penis enhancement chat rooms. But what makes this method a little different is the fact that it is designed only to increase the size of the head. Gripping the base of the penis in one hand, hold firmly enough to trap the blood flow. Then, slowly start moving your hand upwards, pushing the blood to the tip. You should notice the head becoming quite warm and red, and maybe even larger within a single workout. However, the ize will go back to normal within a few minutes of completing the workout, and it will be four or five days before you notice the head size increasing permanently during erections.

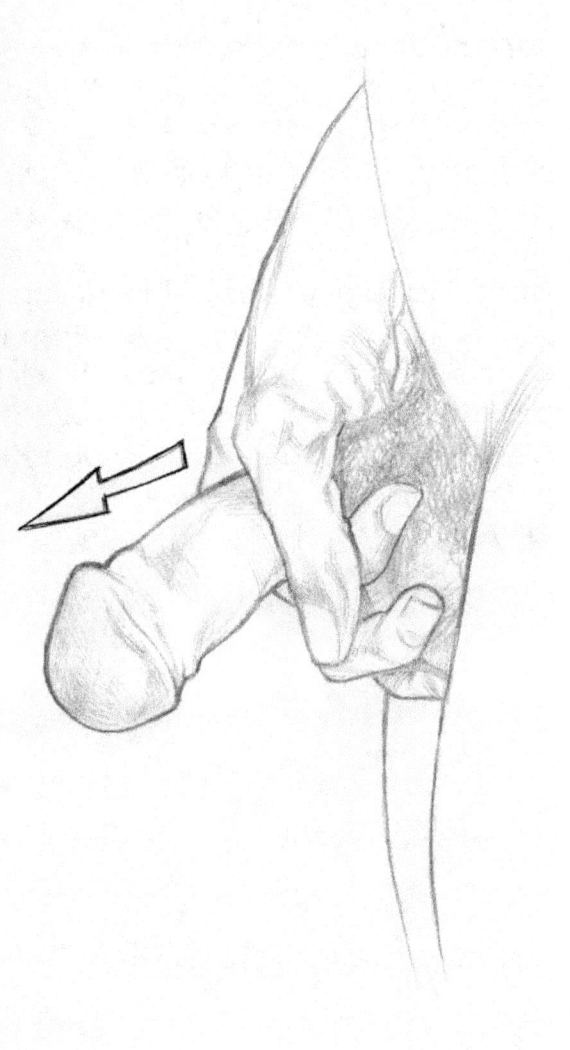

About the 'Dry Method'

If you have heard of jelqing before, you have probably heard of 'doing it dry'. This is more or less exactly what it sounds like. You repeatedly 'milk' the penis with no lubrication whatsoever, holding just as tightly, or tighter to deal with the friction. This doesn't work any better, and, in fact, can actually damage the tissue of the penis. Not to mention it just smarts. Can you imagine repeatedly stroking your penis without anything to ease friction? Even if you still have your foreskin, it will not be a pleasant experience. With you creating so much blood flow, and holding to tightly, tearing can even occur if you are uncut. Trust me on this one, a dry rub isn't the way to go here.

Chapter 6: Stamina Exercises

Getting bigger is all well and good, but even if you managed to jack up your Johnson to a full foot it would mean nothing if you weren't able to last more than a couple of seconds, or, God forbid, couldn't keep it up. But if this is the case, and you have trouble satisfying your partner, you will want to make a large part of your routine's priorities stamina exercises.

If you don't have that problem, you might still want to include these. Stamina exercises are more than just for staying power, despite their name. They are also there for you to increase your own abilities towards pleasure. These workouts will work to give you more frequent erections, make you last longer, intensify your orgasms, and give you harder erections. They will also give you a stronger ejaculate stream.

Use these with the warm up given in Chapter 3. Once you have prepared, you can do these on their own. You can also do them with your others, but they work best if done prior to any length or girth workouts. This is due to the fact that they gets the blood flowing more than any other workout. This will aid you in your size exercises, since the blood will pump more quickly once the tissue is stretched.

One thing to note is that these workouts can be done more than any of the others. There is no real limit on how many of these you can do. In the case of kegels (explained below) it is actually beneficial to do a large number of them through the day. Since they can be done discreetly, you can even practice them in the middle of your office at work, or on the couch when you are watching TV. No one will have any idea, though you might end up getting a bit of a giggle out of it.

Kegels

One of the most common sexual exercises for both men and women, kegels are well known for helping to improve both stamina and endurance. They work by isolating the PC muscles within the groin, which can be flexed to create more control and increase blood flow. It is easy to find this muscle. When you are going to the bathroom, take a moment to stop the flow of urine. The muscles you clench up to do that? That is you PC. You may have also noticed that muscle tensing up just before orgasm; though you may be a little too distracted to notice it then.

Now that you know what it is, you are ready to learn what to do with it. Taking a deep breath, tense the muscle. You should feel your testicles rising up slightly and holding. Keep yourself tense for five seconds, and then slowly release. Remember to be flexing your PC muscles, and not your anus of abdomen. A good rule of thumb: if your balls aren't hopping up, you're doing it wrong. Do these as often as you like, as many times as you like.

Sit Down Wally Ups

Sit Down Wally Ups, also known as Wally Wally Ups, are a popular exercise that are commonly recommended for anyone who wants to strengthen their erection, and increase their ejaculations and orgasms intensity. Please note that you should not do this exercise more than a few times a week, preferably every other day.

Sit down on the edge of a chair so that your testicles are hanging down (not a pretty sight, but necessary). Bring your penis to a full erection, as hard as you can, and make sure to have some kind of stimulation to keep yourself hard throughout. Taking a towel, move it to your penis so that it lays across it, pushing it down as you tightly hold either end. The towel should be taut. Flex your PC muscles, making your penis move upward. Hold for three to five seconds, pushing your penis against the towel, fighting the resistance. Do this for no more than a minute each workout.

Flex Ups

This workout can be done as frequently as desired, just like kegels. It is used to pump up your body's ability to resist orgasm, keeping you from shooting off too early, or just allowing you to control your climax. The idea is to build up resistance by strengthening the muscles of the lower body, including in the anus, the abdomen, and the PC muscles.

Lay down on the floor, knees bent and feet flat. Take a deep breath, then slowly flex your abdominal, PC, and anal muscles, raising yourself up off the ground by your hips. Your upper body should remain firmly on the floor. Hold for five second, then release your breath and lower yourself back down. This should make a thrusting motion, up and down, with your hips. Make sure you are not flexing your thigh muscles, or pushing from your back.

All of these exercises are well known for increasing stamina, endurance, and pleasure. The first and third workout can even more for women to tighten the vaginal muscles and intensify their orgasms. Just to give you a little hint if you have a wife who might be interested in joining you in this little journey.

Chapter 7: The Warm Up Phase

You can come up with your very own routine that will meet your needs. However, there are a few tried and true methods that will get help you through the three phases of penile growth. The first of these phases is The Warm Up Phase. This is when you first begin to stretch out the tissue of the penile, and gain stamina. The thing to keep in mind is that you will rarely see any but the most minimal results. However, it is the most important phase out of the three, as it prepares for the greater growths in the second phase.

If you want improve in all ways when it comes to your penis, the best thing you can do is follow this Warm Up routine, and then go from there. Once you have started to see some results, you can make variations that will aim more towards whatever the main adjustments you are looking to make. You can also keep to this routine the whole way through, until you are ready to move into phase two.

The Routine

Start out by slowly arousing yourself to semi-erect, making sure you are in a warm room. Remember that doing this in the shower is often best, but if not you should have lubricant at the ready, as well as anything else you might need, like a warm bowl of water. Once you have managed all of this, you are good to go.

1. Power Stretch – Do the Power Stretch for two full minutes, making sure to use plenty of lubrication. Keep in mind that the first time you do this could be aggravating to your penis. Try to create as little friction as possible when you perform the Power Stretch, and never do it for longer than the two minutes you first week.

2. Circular Stretch – Do the Circular Stretch for three full minutes, and the same amount of lubrication should be applied. This stretch can cause more irritating than the Power Stretch, as you will be moving your shaft in circles. Using your thumb and forefinger, instead of a full fist, will reduce the rubbing. But you have to hold tighter to do it this way, so make sure you have a tight hold. Unlike the power stretch, letting go might not just send you back into place. You will be making circular motions, and so a sudden drop can actually sprain your penis if you were gripping too hard, or moving too fast.

3. Jelq 1, 2, or 3 – You can do any one of these Jelqs as a part of your Warm Up routine. However, you should only use one until you move into the second phase. This is to keep from causing irritation to the shaft of the penis, which will become rather sore if you start out using more than one. Perform your chosen jelq for a full three minutes, or four if you are not feeling too sore by the end of it. Do not exceed this amount, and only do the Jelqs every other day.

4. Stamina Exercises – Do as many of these, and as often, as you like. Remember, workouts to increase stamina and endurance can only help you, and can be done separately from the others. Make sure to do these every day. To test how they are working, test your urine stream, You should be able to more quickly and easily cut off the stream as time goes on. You will also begin to see yourself becoming erect more easily and quickly, so save it until the end, when you don't have to be soft or semi-erect.

How do I Know I'm Ready for Phase Two?

It will be fairly obvious when you are ready to move into the next phase of routines, because you will begin to see some results. I don't mean you will wake up one day and barely be able to lift your leg because of the size of you schlong – keep dreaming!

– but you should see a portion of an inch of growth and some girth increases. This takes about four or five days for most, but some might end up seeing it in as little as two or three. This will usually depend on your starting point, and the size you are when you are erect.

Can I Stay with the Warm Up Phase for Longer?

Yes, you can keep going with this phase for as long as you like, but keep in mind that the longer you stay with it past seeing results, the less they will work. For some, it may take seven to ten days to move on, or to feel confident enough that they have made the progress to move on. This will be a matter of personal preference, and you will have to judge for yourself where you are. If it takes longer don't feel discouraged; it doesn't mean there is anything wrong with your junk. You are just a slightly late bloomer, as it were.

Can I Skip the Warm Up Phase?

Yes, but I wouldn't recommend it. Your penis will need time to adjust to what is being done. You need to begin the first stages of stretching the tissue, and moving too quickly can actually cause damage. This might hinder your progress, and even cause some pain. The last thing you will want to tell your partner is that you can't get it on because you hurt yourself trying to jack up your Johnson.

Once you have moved beyond this point, and you have started to see results, you are ready to move onto phase two, or the Active Phase. This is where you will begin to see real results, and at a much faster rate. This is the part where you will usually end up where you want to be, within the first seven to ten days. Let's get started, and get that penis into gear!

Chapter 8: The Active Phase

Congratulations! If you have reached the active phase you have already been seeing some results from your daily exercises, and you are quite aware of a number of the techniques, and how it is that they work. From here on the results should be more palpable, from stamina to performance. This is the phase that this entire book is all about, and likely what you have been waiting for.

The thing about this phase is that there is very little by way of routine that will work more than any other. It will all become a matter of building it up based on what it is you want to work on most, and focusing your time on that. If you want to work on both length and girth you will want to split it up to work on both for the maximum amount of time that you can safely do it.

The best way to go about it is to try everything provided in this book that is within the category you want to work on. I don't mean do every single one each day you do your workouts, though I suppose you could if you felt like it. I mean just taking the first day to try them all out, and find which ones work more naturally for you.

It is important that you do not do any of the exercises that feel unnatural, uncomfortable, or painful. None of these should be very difficult, and while they may feel a little odd, they should never hurt. If they do, you should stop immediately. If it hurts to turn your penis in any one direction, you will want to see a doctor. This could be due to a condition called Peyronie's disease, which is a severe curvature of the penis. While the stretching workouts in this book can help correct some of the curve in your junk, it won't cure a disease. You will need a doc if it gets bad.

Working Out a Routine

Working on your active phase routine should, ideally, start from the method mentioned above. Take the first day and try out each exercise offered in chapters four, five, and six. Find out which ones you prefer, and which ones you would prefer not to use. This could be because they are painful, you don't like the movement, or they just didn't do it for you in the Warm Up Phase.

Write down each one you want to use, and once you have a general list, start to work out how many reps you want to do, for how long. Keep in mind that you will want to keep your routine between ten and fifteen minutes, never more, and never less. This is only for length and girth workouts...all stamina exercises can be done as many times as you like, and separately.

To find the time that you allot to each workout should depend on what you want to work on more. Let's say that you want to work more on length than girth, but want to work on girth as well, and you have decided on a full fifteen minute workout system. Rather than split it evenly, you would add a few more minutes to the side of length. So, length might be nine minutes, while girth around six minutes.

If you want to work on both evenly, you would just split it right down the middle. Just remember to work that time in so that you evenly distribute the time between each exercise within that window. None of them work any better than the others, exactly. It will be more of a matter of preference, comfort, and occasionally a difference in the tissue within the penis, and how it responds to certain movements and blood flow.

Can I See an Example?

OK, here is an example of a common workout routine so that all of you nervous blokes that still worry about doing it wrong can see. This is a routine used by one of the men who used my routine. He started out with 5 ½ inches long, and a circumference of 4 inches (both while erect). His ending results were 7 ¼ inches long, and a circumference of 5 inches.

Mike's Routine:

- 3 minutes Power Stretch

- 3 minutes V Stretch

- 3 minutes Circular Stretch

- 2 minutes Jelq Form 2

- 2 minutes Jelq Form 3

- 2 minutes Jelq Form 4

- 10 minutes kegals

- 10 minutes Sit Down Wally Ups

- 5 minutes Flex Ups

When Do I Know I'm Done with This Phase?

This is not always easy to tell. For some people they will stop growing completely, and no matter how much they work they will see no further gains. Some will just begin to slow down, and so they will be forced to recognize that their Active Phase is coming to an end. Still others will just see the results they want, and see no need to go further.

Chapter 9: The Plateau Phase

By now you will have seen a great deal of progress. You have probably been at it for a week, maybe two, and while you say serious improvements up until this point, those improvements have started to slow. They may have ever stopped completely, and no matter how many times you stretch, pull, and metaphorically beat your penis into submission it just refuses to lurch forward another fraction of an inch.

This is what we in the dick business call 'The Plateau Phase'. It happens with all workouts, no matter what area you are trying to improve. Those losing weight will notice the rate of their weight loss deteriorate. When people are bulking up we'll see a slowing of growth in muscle mass. Those trying to gain weight might see that the scale just refuses to go up. This is frustrating, sometimes maddening, but perfectly normal and even has a name: diminishing returns.

I wish I could tell you that, like the other examples, it fades and your junk will start to expand with a shift in workout. Sometimes, when you have only slowed and not stopped, this is the case. But chances are you have reached your limit. Your penis is a sensitive thing, much more than even the most paranoid ball-defenders often realize. The tissues can only stretch so far, and only so much blood can be held within its' chambers. It is generally at this point you should through in the towel, and be happy for the blessings that have so far been bestowed on you.

But What if I Have Only Slowed?

For some, the journey may not yet be over. Your progress may not have stopped dead, but instead slowed significantly. When this happens, you will want to change your workout. Start adding more frequency to some exercises, switch others out with another, and chance the time of reps for all of it. Take it easy for a few days and start again, just like you would with any other kind of plateau. From there you should start building slowly again.

What if I Start to Lose My Gains?

This shouldn't happen too much, but some might start to see their numbers go down again. This is an opportunity for you to start again, and start building it back up. Sometimes with this slow build you can even get greater numbers that before, with slightly variations in the routine. Not everyone will be able to do this, however, and they will need to add in some of the stamina routines on a long term basis to keep circulation moving.

Can I Keep Using Them Anyway?

For most, I wouldn't recommend it. It is like any workout, if you push too hard you will hurt yourself. The only exercises you should keep doing are those meant for stamina, specifically kegels. These workouts are always great, and for a multitude of reasons. Feel free to keep them up as long as you like, without waning. This will help you with your stamina and endurance in the long term, and may even give you total control over your erections and orgasms.

But I Don't Want to Stop!

Tough. You have two options here. Stop, and be grateful for the increases in size and girth you have established, or yank the tissue out of place and cause tearing trying to squeeze a little more juice from the lemon. Of course, it is your choice. But have you ever heard the phrase "Don't look a gift horse in the mouth?" Well, in this case it would be "Don't look a gift penis in the head." Be happy with what you have, and move on.

Chapter 9: Other Factors to Maximize Fitness

There are a number of things that can actually affect the size of your penis, and even more that can affect the performance. There are also a number of other methods that have been created to help men just like you jack up their size. But how important are these facts, and how helpful are these other methods? Each has a different level of what is and isn't helpful, and we will look at several of the most commonly asked about items on the 'Penis Size' list now.

Diet

Believe it or not, this is a big one. What you eat will affect your body in a multitude of ways, from the way you sleep, to the weight that you gain. But one of the lesser known side effects of a bad diet is penis shrinkage. That's right, fellas, your old boy can shrink up a few inches when you put the wrong foods in your mouth. Numerous studies have been done to confirm this fact, and even the American Medical Association recommends certain foods be avoided.

Junk Food That Hurts Your Junk:

• White bread

- White pasta

- White rice

- Foods with empty carbs

- Anything fried

- Anything high in fat

- Red meat

- High-sugar foods

- High-sodium foods

All of this should be a no-brainer, right? And yet, these commonly eaten food items are some of the most eaten in the West. This means a number of health issues have crept up in recent years, and as a consequence, the dong has suffered. High blood pressure and cholesterol can limit the amount of blood flow that gets down there, which can create less frequent erections that are less hard, and less powerful. It also shrinks them down a great deal.

An excess of fat can also create problems for those of you who carry it around the belly. This is the most common way that men carry their weight, and while it doesn't make the penis smaller, it will make it harder to get to the whole of it. The base will be further back, with the fat keeping the depth you are able to go during sex. This effectively eliminates a portion of your size, which is a big problem for your partner.

Food That Loves Your Junk:

• Fish

• Peanuts, almonds, or anything high in Omega-3 fatty acids

• Chicken

• Citrus

• Whole wheat and grains

• Any vegetables

Exercise

We have already covered how excess weight can really cause a droop in your penis. Therefore, it stands to reason that a workout will be an important part of your daily health routine. Not only will this push down blood pressure and cholesterol by burning calories and fat, but it will give you added energy as well. It will also improve circulation, and since you need proper blood flow to get your general standing to attention, this is obviously needed.

There is another benefit to regular exercise, however. That is the relief of heavy stress, which can be a huge factor in stamina and endurance. Just think of the last time you were under a huge amount of stress...how did the jimmy work? Probably not so well, if you could even get it up. Getting rid of some of that tension in some intensive cardio will do your penis some good, and will make you feel better in general.

Pills, Pumps, and Extenders

These are useless. Really, they are, I have not seen a single one that has been worth the money. Some have even been significantly dangerous. While the pumps may seem like they work they will only draw a little more blood for a short time. Extenders can tear the tissue, and should be avoided at all costs. Pills can be potentially dangerous, and most are just pointless herbs thrown into a capsule, and would go better on a salad than in a penile enhancement product.

In the end, you are almost certainly not going to find anything that will be worth buying within this genre. If you find something that works, please feel free to contact me and let me know. I would be happy to take the time to test it, research it, and add it into another edition. But my hopes are not high, and I certainly believe that is it the methods given in this book that will get you to your goals, not those promised by marketing companies.

Surgery

When all else fails, there is always surgery. However, this method is extremely dangerous, rarely works to more than a fraction of an inch, and is usually only given to those with a significant problem. This means well under the average, such as three inches when erect. Surgery is also occasionally used for severe curvatures that cause main during sexual activity with a partner. It is not just given to anyone who decides they want to widdle a few inches onto their wang.

There are a number of risks involved with this procedure. Infections are a big one, as they do require some cutting to be done. The cutting should be a deterrent on its' own...do you really want a scalpel jockey waving a blade down there? Another risk is loss of sensitivity, and occasionally impotence. You can actually affect your ability to get an erection without using medication.

Prescription Medication

Finally, we have prescription drugs. These will not increase size, but they can improve performance. But they are meant for people who have real problems getting it up, a problem that comes with high blood pressure, age, intense and recurrent anxiety, and a number of serious health issues. You should never take these pills for recreation, or without needing them. While it isn't clear what could happen (not enough studies have been done), there have been cases of it mixing badly without other drugs and causing stroke and heart failure. You don't want to kick the bucket while you're kicking boots.

At this point, you might be seeing the problem with penile enlargement. I have been in the business a long time, and seen a lot of things. I have used plenty of things as well, and I can tell you that natural exercises are the way to go. They are safe, effective, and cause no long term damage. Stick with what works, and stay away from the ridiculous ideas posted on the Internet.

Chapter 10: Afterword

We have discussed just about every aspect of penile fitness in the last few chapters. We have covered the ways to improve penile performance, the science behind increasing it, and how to do so. We have talked about what does and doesn't work, and how to handle each phase of your journey. I have made endless penis-related jokes, and used a number of euphemisms that has had the effect of amusing me throughout the creation of this book. But there is one thing that we have not really spoken about, and that is your own, personal view on penis size, which is really at the heart of this.

I know as a guy that this is a sensitive issue for all of us. We see the size of our penis as a testament to our very manhood, more than just our ability to satisfy a lover. But again, this comes with its own set of problems. When we feel inadequate, we can project our dissatisfaction with whatever to an organ that often has nothing to do with it. The purpose behind this book is not to convince you that you have to pump it up, or that a big shlong is the best relationship advice.

While you will likely have your reasons for working on your lower regions, just keep in mind that whatever anxiety you feel is probably one-sided, and that it is doubtful that your partner feels the same. Most women complain about 'too big', and rarely do you hear 'too small'. If you are to worry about size, be sure you are doing it for the right reasons. Let it be a personal goal, and not something you feel should make or break your relationship, whether potential or an existing one.

Remember, whether you are in a long term relationship or just having fun, your penis is just another tool in this game of life. There are a billion of ways to please a woman (whether sexually or not) and your penis is just one of them. But in the end, regardless of your goals, I hope you find someone who values you not only for your excellently performing penis but also for who you are as a person. That, my friend, is the best recipe for happiness, sexual or otherwise.

Now don't get too sentimental, better run out to get some lube, you've got work to do. Seriously though, this book should help you improve your sexual performance, but remember, your penis is just another part of the painting, don't lose sight of the rest!

Until next time, good luck, and good penis health.

www.ingramcontent.com/pod-product-compliance
Lightning Source LLC
Chambersburg PA
CBHW062109280526
45788CB00003B/1411